YOUR KID AND CROHN'S

A Parent's Handbook

William Sparke

APS BOOKS
STOURBRIDGE

Your Kid and Crohn's: A Parent's Handbook
Copyright ©2015 APS Publications

All rights reserved.
The moral right of the author William Sparke has been asserted.

No part of this publication may be reproduced, stored in or introduced into a retrieval system, or transmitted, in any form, or by any means (electronic, mechanical, photocopying, recording or otherwise) without the written permission of the publisher except that brief selections may be quoted or copied without permission, provided that full credit is given.

APS Publications,
4 Oakleigh Road,
Stourbridge,
West Midlands,
DY8 2JX

www.andrewsparke.com

CONTENTS

First Thoughts ~ 1
Diagnosis and Despair ~ 2
Symptoms ~ 5
Falling Ill ~ 10
    Bathrooms
    Food
    Hospital Time
Lifestyle Issues ~ 15
    School
    School Toilets
    Social Anxiety
    Motivation
    Embarrassment
Friends and Family ~ 18
Medical Issues ~ 20
    Blood Tests and Needles
    Colonoscopy
    Barium X-Rays
    Wireless Capsule Endoscopy
    MRE and CT Scans
    Ultrasound
    Medication
    Steroids
    Liquid Diets
    Further Treatment
    Biological Therapies
    Surgery
Compromising To Live ~ 37
Holistic Symptom Management ~ 39
Closing Comments On Nutrition ~ 40

Key Terms ~ 41
Further Information ~ 42

FIRST THOUGHTS

As I enter the final year of my undergraduate degree I have found myself achieving just exactly what I wanted from my life at this point and I note that I am holding my own in relation to my peers. This might not sound like the loftiest of goals for a 24 year old but I am proud of where I am. The road has been a lot more difficult than it could have been. This is where the idea for writing this guide comes from. As someone diagnosed with Crohn's Disease at nine years of age, I have realised that I have some insights that can help others travelling the same road. I want to help you and your child get through a life changing event and give you some tips on how to adapt, how to cope and then how to thrive.

Surprisingly enough I feel that, alongside the dark times, Crohn's has left me with some of the best memories I have as well as some of the closest relationships of anyone I know. I guess I've come to conclude that in some regards this curse has been a bit of a blessing.

DIAGNOSIS AND DESPAIR

It is my understanding that, at just nine years old, I was diagnosed very young. But in a lot of respects everything surrounding my diagnosis was conspicuously lucky. To start with I was diagnosed within one month of first falling ill. Probably a record for Crohn's. Initially I presented with all of the standard symptoms of a pretty nasty stomach bug. I had stopped eating and was going to the toilet fifteen or more times a day and so was sent home from the GP with some Imodium and the friendly advice to my mother that I would be fine in a few days. Two weeks down the line I was still most definitely not fine, and was now in severe discomfort verging on pain. To top it all off I was beginning to lose weight quickly.

Having never been a particularly robust or large child this obviously had my parents incredibly worried. Fortunately, instead of spending the next few months or even years bouncing between GP's looking for answers, as I am well aware can happen, my GP immediately referred me to a specialist team dedicated to treating children with Crohn's Disease and I passed into the care of the Royal Free Hospital in London. He did this for one simple reason. Two of his own children had Crohn's and he recognised the pattern. What were the odds of that I wonder?

I was seen the next day, had a barrage of tests done and by the end of the week I had my diagnosis. I was nine years old, I had Crohn's disease and my life had just changed. After the doctors were done talking, explaining the situation, explaining the illness, explaining their plans for how to treat me and explaining how my life was going to change, the first thing I remember was crying. Not so much at the diagnosis. To be honest that was quite a relief. To know what is going on and that there are people who think they can help is no small thing and goes a long way to making a situation more bearable. I cried because I was tired and I felt terrible. As far as I was concerned I had just had the worst few days of my life. In short I wanted to go home and I wanted this to be happening to someone else. On top of everything else I wanted a cheese-burger. After those two days of tests I wanted a cheeseburger more than anything in the world. But between a liquid diet and a slow reintroduction to solid food I would have to wait more than 3 months for that burger. There's nothing like suffering and deprivation to make a treat worthwhile. I remember every detail. It was the best burger I have eaten in my life!

Those few days of tests and two months of being on a liquid diet taught me a lot about myself. But the most important lesson I would want to pass on is that although you cannot choose the situation, you most definitely can choose how you and the people around you approach it, and this is what we found ourselves doing rather than lingering in denial.

As a family we threw ourselves into the situation with the gusto of a group possessed and as a result, what could have been traumatic childhood memories blossomed into treasured family memories. Every day trip to the hospital became an opportunity to search for silver linings in obscure places, be these an opportunity to have lunch with my gran before we went in for a blood test, or a trip to the book shop with my mum so that I would have a book to read while I sat in the waiting room, or something I wouldn't have dreamed of finding or seeing in London. My family were great at turning those days from something most people would want to forget into something I will always remember.

Over the past fourteen years I have experienced more different medications and treatment plans than I can possibly recall, name or fully evaluate in detail. Some of them have worked and some of them have not. More frustratingly though, some of the have worked for some time before either an intolerance to them developed or the disease just regressed. And this is one of the key problems of Crohn's; it's very inconsistency. The disease goes into remission for indeterminate amounts of time. During these periods everything is good and you are healthy. However at the back of your mind there is always the knowledge that although you are perfectly well today, you might not be so tomorrow. This unpredictability can make Crohn's hard for the uninformed observer to understand, and it is something that your child will be likely to come to know only too well so don't forget it.

That's not to say that you should let them live in fear of the disease resurging. Instead just be there for them and be understanding when it happens. The timing might never be other than inconvenient but there is not really anything that can be done about that. As I said earlier, you can't control the disease only how you address the situation and this is the key lesson to pass on to your child.

SYMPTOMS

The symptoms of Crohn's Disease can vary from the merely unpleasant to the downright painful and can vary pretty much from case to case depending on which part of the digestive system is inflamed. Fortunately no one knows your child like you do, so most of the symptoms should be easy enough to spot if you know what you're looking for. From there it's just a case of mitigating these as best you can in order to help the child lead as normal of a life as possible.

Firstly I'll cover the most common symptoms of Crohn's and some of the problems they can present. Number one is the most noticeable symptom to pretty much everyone and this is recurring diarrhoea. Initially this can just look like a stomach bug or mild food poisoning but the key difference is that it either does not go away or recurs regularly. This can obviously be pretty depressing for the person experiencing it, especially if it goes a long time without a cause being diagnosed. Furthermore there are a whole host of other potential problems that can be brought to the fore by having recurring diarrhoea. Some of these are more obvious and easier to address.

One tip I can give you is to invest in toilet wipes infused with aloe vera and also quilted toilet paper. Since your child is using the bathroom a lot, regular toilet paper can rapidly begin to feel like sandpaper, leaving the affected area sore and inflamed. This is both painful and embarrassing so, if you can, head it off before it becomes an issue.

The next common symptom we are going to discuss is abdominal pain and cramping, usually worse after eating. This can vary from some mild discomfort to complete agony. One of the key complications I have found from this is that it can really mess up the way a person views food. This in turn will often lead to the sufferer, both consciously and subconsciously, trying to avoid food as much as possible. As a parent it is obviously distressing to see your child not eating and it can lead to arguments as the stress of the situation begins to wear on family relationships.

As a parent the key traits you will need to exhibit are patience and understanding. It is not the child's fault that he or she is turning down the food you are offering and, if asked for alternatives, the child may be unable to suggest any that would please them. Alternatively they may offer suggestions in order to appease you or just try to find something and then go on to not eat them. While I appreciate that this can be very frustrating, you need to remember that for a child with Crohn's food can be a very confusing subject. This is particularly true as abdominal pain and cramping can combine with some of the other symptoms to turn food, from a source of nutrition and enjoyment, into a source of pain to be shunned and avoided whenever possible.

Another of the most common symptoms that is present with Crohn's disease is extreme tiredness, more commonly referred to as fatigue. This is probably one of the easiest symptoms for you to understand having undoubtedly, as a parent, experienced feeling so tired that you can feel you can't move or so exhausted that the smallest task feels like climbing a mountain. For your child this is what they probably feel like a lot of the time especially when they are actively experiencing a flare up and the disease is not in remission. Again, as with the abdominal pain and cramping, the best thing you can do is be patient and understanding. As a side note it's worth remembering that we all get a bit short tempered and snappy when we are shattered, so if you are finding your child arguing more than usual remember that it is in no way personally directed at you. Most likely the child is just lashing out as a result of confusion and exhaustion. Looking back I certainly did. This has left me feeling quite lucky that everyone around me was so understanding and supportive of this.

The next of the most common symptoms of Crohn's Disease is unexplained and sometimes substantial weight loss. Fortunately as a parent this will probably be pretty evident to you since it is likely that no one is paying more attention to your child than you are. Not that this makes it any easier for you to deal with, but catching stuff like this early can make a difference. Getting treatment earlier will hopefully prevent too much weight being lost. Obviously this is better for your child's health and overall development.

The last of the most common symptoms that presents in most cases of Crohn's Disease, is the presence of blood and mucus in the child's faeces (stools, poop - use whatever term you like). Now this is one of the harder symptoms for you to spot as a parent unless the child is concerned about the change and actively comes and asks you. My advice here would be that if your child has one or more of the other symptoms of Crohn's, take the initiative to check for yourself if blood or mucus is present before they flush the toilet. Obviously this can be a slightly odd thing for you to request, but this is really a symptom you don't want to be left unaware of as it's a big warning sign.

You may find that some of these symptoms described above are intermittent, coming and going for a period of weeks or months at a time. These periods of relative health are known as remission and they can usually be followed by periods of being ill (or flare ups). As such the standard medical advice given by the NHS is that if your child has one or more of these problems which are persisting or recurring you should take your child to see your GP and bring up the possibility of Crohn's disease.

There are also several less other common symptoms of Crohn's Disease.

Firstly we have a persisting high fever of 38 degrees C (100 degrees F) or above, this is obviously pretty uncomfortable and will contribute to your child's overall sensation of feeling ill.

Secondly we have the potentially unending nausea, the feeling that you are about to be sick. This is obviously very unpleasant for the sufferer and sadly there is not really a whole lot you as a parent can do to help. What you can do however is to understand how this symptom can enhance the tendency to avoid food as much as possible as discussed earlier when looking some of the more common symptoms of Crohn's. At this point hopefully you can begin to see how the whole topic of food could rapidly become more trouble than its worth in a child's mind. Diarrhoea cramps and pain followed by potentially being sick, or at least the feeling that you are likely to be; these are the things that become associated with food and eating in general.

Next up we have joint pain and swelling, akin to arthritis. Fortunately not all sufferers of Crohn's experience this but for those who do it's obviously very uncomfortable or painful. This is probably one of the most frustrating symptoms for a child, particularly an active one. A lot of your child's favourite activities suddenly have become beyond them. Love playing sports? Can't because your knees hurt if you run too far now. Love playing on the computer? Can't do that all day anymore because your hands hurt. This can quickly become very depressing and frustrating and you need to watch out for this.

The next symptom of note is the presence of mouth ulcers. These are very uncomfortable, sometimes painful and pretty much guaranteed to be irritated by putting any food in your mouth. The only way to address these as far as I am aware is getting medical treatment to control the Crohn's Disease. Piecemeal solutions are at best short-term palliatives.

It is probably also worth noting that children with Crohn's disease may grow at a slower rate and so may be smaller than their classmates. This is due to the inflammation caused by the disease in the gut preventing the body absorbing nutrients from any food you can actually get them to eat.

An occasional but hugely distressing symptom of Crohn's arises from stomach cramping and small sections of inflamed intestine sticking together. This can happen in the rectal area and if the bowel wall sticks together at this point it can lead to the creation of a small sore open to the outside from which excreta can leak. This is known as a fistula. It will seldom if ever go away or heal of its own accord, however much antiseptic you apply. Please consult your GP as soon as possible because minor surgical intervention can resolve a fistula before it becomes an entrenched and painful problem.

There are other symptoms associated with Crohn's which may at first seem unrelated because they are nothing to do with the digestive system. The form of arthritis already mentioned is one such. Another is a tendency towards dryness of the eyes. One of the final symptoms you may notice is that your child's lips may become very dry, cracking in a painful manner that can lead to sores around the corners of their mouth. If left untreated these can become infected, leaving them both painful and unsightly.

FALLING ILL

The initial stages of falling ill with Crohn's disease is often described as one of the hardest and emotionally draining parts of the whole sorry business. There are many factors which can contribute to this. Particularly for a child this time is very hard and not just because of the symptoms themselves but also due to the psychological response.

The person experiencing the symptoms won't forget about them, even in remission, and neither should you. That is not to say that you should spend all your time worrying about where the nearest bathroom is or when they last ate. Instead it is just something to keep in mind. The lack of a definitive explanation of what is actually going on and why it is happening will also be weighing heavily on the mind of the child. This can of itself be both distressing and depressing. So clarifying what symptoms have been and are still occurring is vital. Communication with your child is all. They must not be allowed to clam up and bear their symptoms in silence.

In this section I'm going to lay out some of the problems that are commonly encountered in between the periods of first falling ill, getting a diagnosis and finally beginning treatment. It is important to remember that this will most likely be a time of considerable change and acclimatisation for both you and the child. So I'll be examining some of the physical issues which your child is likely to face and examining some tips and tricks to help you handle them.

Bathrooms

Unfortunately if you have Crohn's disease you are going to become very familiar with the bathroom. The nature of the illness sort of demands it. To understand the growing and complicated relationship your child now has with the bathroom it is necessary to put yourself into their shoes and understand their thought processes. Firstly you need to understand that with Crohn's you feel the need to go to the toilet a lot of the time, even when you don't need to. This is obviously very uncomfortable. You know that sensation of really needing to go to the loo. Well your child is probably experiencing that 24 hours a day. Imagine that for a moment and you can begin to see that this will affect how your child is both consciously and subconsciously structuring their day.

For them the need to be near a toilet is a necessity. This may even make them somewhat reclusive as they shy away from situations which put uncertain variables into place. Variables such as where is the nearest bathroom? Will I be able to get to the bathroom if I need to? These are the sorts of questions which can dominate the mind of a young person suffering from Crohn's.

Fortunately however this is something that you as a parent can address or at least help with. Indeed a little forward planning can to a certain extent neutralize this issue. As a parent if you always know where the nearest toilet is it will go a long way to helping your kid feel comfortable. Knowing that there is someone else who knows, who understands and more importantly is looking out for them in this particular if somewhat peculiar way. The knowledge that if they say they need the toilet, the request will be treated with a certain sense of urgency which is often denied to young children. This can particularly be the case in a classroom environment. It might be a good idea to have a quiet word with your child's teacher and filling them in on the situation, making the classroom a much less scary place.

This next tip might seem like a little bit of a no-brainer but if you could always have a pack of tissues on you at all times that would be great. Just in case there isn't any loo-roll wherever you happen to find yourselves. This might sound strange but there are few things less funny than finding no toilet paper in a place that's not home.

Food

Food and your child's eating habits are possibly one of the hardest areas for any parent to deal with when it comes to your kid and Crohn's Disease. The fact of the matter is that your child's relationship with food has probably just changed to something so alien to you that it likely baffles and confuses you. This is something that is probably going to frustrate you a lot and you are going to have to come to terms with it. In order to gain the necessary understanding you'll have to examine how your child now feels about food and really views the whole nutrition process.

Firstly let's discuss the experience of eating for someone with Crohn's disease and then we can begin to break down some of the thought processes beginning to become associated with eating and with food in general. It is necessary for any parent to understand that for a child with Crohn's eating quickly becomes associated with a whole host of bad things, starting with indigestion and stomach cramps and with the less than reassuring knowledge that eating may leave you feeling a lot worse than you already did. In essence food can quickly become associated with the symptoms of the illness, hardly an illogical conclusion for a child to make and so naturally they may end up trying to avoid food as much as possible.

Choosing to avoid food is obviously a bit of a catch-22 when losing weight and is something that you will want to avoid for your child. As such one of the best things you can do is listen to them when they are telling you what kinds of food can work for them.

Hospital Time

All of you are now going to get very familiar with both inpatient and outpatient proceedings but fortunately this is one of your best opportunities to create good memories and find silver linings. Here we shall examine some potential ways to turn these days out into good times.

One of the first ways to do this is to look for an opportunity for a nice lunch or breakfast together. This can be a bonding time and instead of being apprehensive about hospital time the child can look forward to his or her time out with you.

Another good idea here is to get your family involved as much as possible. Apart from giving you a much needed break this will allow your child to look forward to different days out with different family members. This helps to ensure that your child not only feels like they have lots of people who understand and are on their side, but over time will hopefully help them move from being apprehensive about hospital days to actively looking forward to them.

My second key tip is to learn the names of everyone you see, the doctors, and the nurses and even the secretaries. While you're doing this make sure that they know who you are too. Take a pen and paper with you and list the names of everyone involved in the treatment process and what their job is. This will make it a lot easier for you to chase up the appropriate people if you feel that anything is being mishandled or there is something you're not happy with.

Finally always chase things up. Don't be afraid to call people up if you feel that there are unnecessary delays or if you feel you are not being given enough priority. It may surprise you to know that the wheels of bureaucracy will turn a lot quicker if everyone inside the system knows that not only have you called them three times today, but you will politely and insistently do so tomorrow and the day after that until you get the results you need.

LIFESTYLE ISSUES

I am now going to discuss some of the most common difficulties which can affect a child with Crohn's Disease and how you can help to manage some of these. First up is the need to maintain social relationships during a flare up and how this can be difficult for your child.

School:
When it comes to school-work the fact of the matter is that you could be looking at an uphill struggle. The message you have to sell is that studying may well be harder while coping with the symptoms of Crohn's but it will be worth it in the end. The key lesson to pass on is that there is no substitute for hard work, no matter how much potential and talent is present. For a young person with Crohn's Disease this is particularly true. The fact of the matter is that a lot of this period in your child's life is going to be harder than for other children not least because of the other obstacles they are facing and concerns they are dealing with that their friends don't have.

School toilets:

This is something you can address and do something about. As you most likely remember from your own schooldays, in a school environment you are not in control of when you can go to the bathroom. Instead you must wait for the teacher to give you permission to leave the classroom or even be required to wait for another student to go and come back. For someone with Crohn's this is unacceptable. To put it simply, "When you got to go, you really got to go". This is even more true for a child with Crohn's Disease than for anyone else in that classroom. At the same time there are elements of social anxiety that can creep into this situation. How is a child to explain how badly and urgently they need the toilet in a classroom situation? There is pretty much no way for that not to be seriously embarrassing. It would be a very good idea for you to get into contact with your child's school and make sure all of their teachers are aware of the situation. A system needs to be in place that allows the child to leave the classroom whenever they need the bathroom. More importantly the child needs to feel in control of this.

Social Anxiety:

Whether they are worrying about looking obviously ill or being concerned about where the nearest toilet is and if they will be able to reach it; there are plenty of opportunities for things to go embarrassingly wrong in your child's eyes. This is difficult to address to be honest and it something that your child is going to have to learn to deal with over time. Experience has taught me that there is no real substitute for experience in this area and you need to remember that the longer the sufferer has this illness the better they will get at managing these variables. The early days will be difficult but just reassure your child that it will get easier.

Motivation:

The fact of the matter is that when so much is going on in a child's life, school-work can pretty quickly begin to seem less important to them. This is where responsibility falls on your shoulders. As the parent, you, rather than their teachers who will not largely have the time or incentive to concentrate on your child's particular needs, are going to be the sole difference between whether they fall behind and struggle or whether they excel. I cannot stress this enough. You need to be on top of this! You need to be in touch with the school regularly to find out what work is being missed and make sure your child stays reasonably up to date. This will make the transition back into normal education a lot easier when they are healthy again. Once the child falls behind it will be very difficult to catch up as the work will just keep stacking up. You can lose whole years of school this way if you are not careful and nobody wants to be resitting a school year with younger children than themselves.

Embarrassment:

I have focussed at length on the fact that Crohn's and some of its associated symptoms can potentially be very embarrassing so my advice would be to encourage your child to be as open as possible with the people around them and especially with their friends. It is very helpful to have people around you who understand what you are going through and this is no different for your child. Furthermore once the child has people in place who they feel know what is going on and what they are going through, it can greatly help with the social anxiety they are bound to find themselves experiencing.

FRIENDS AND FAMILY

For a person suffering with Crohn's disease, be they an adult or a child, it is very easy to slip into a very antisocial lifestyle. This can be due to a culmination of factors which the sufferer is experiencing, to the fore of which is likely to be the fatigue they are encountering. I will try to help you understand how this can shape how your child goes about planning their life.

Activities can quickly begin to feel like they are more hassle than they are worth. "Even if I go I will be too tired to enjoy it" or "It all just sounds like too much - I'm not sure I can manage that". These are common thoughts for someone who has Crohn's Disease particularly whilst experiencing a flare up and as a parent you need to be aware of this. Then from not wanting to get in a car as it makes them feel sick, thoughts turn to "If we go out will there be a toilet?" And those are just the main objections to going out. A poorly child can find plenty more apparently legitimate reasons to stay at home.

Upon seeing this change in me, one of the best things I feel my parents did was to ensure that I had somewhere to hang out at home where I could have friends over. A play room that later grew into a games-room and finally a den. Throughout my whole childhood, my mum went out of her way to invite other children over as often as possible and this allowed me to retain some semblance of a normal social life and made integrating back into school when I was healthy so much easier. After all I would be joining my friends at school and I already saw those people all the time. I have to say I am so grateful to my parents for that and I would strongly recommend that you approach this problem in the same way.

The next thing you can do to help is bring in the family. By this what I mean is to get your extended family involved as much as possible. Having more people aware of what's going on will not only help your child but there will be additional knock on beneficial effects for both of you. For starters having the rest of your family involved and taking a supportive role will take a substantial amount of the burden off your shoulders. Having someone who understands the situation is not just good for your child but great for you too. Family can also assist with helping you schedule your time at the hospital or when your child is too ill for school. It will also help you keep some semblance of normality in your own life, prevent you becoming isolated and if desired help you to maintain your employment. Furthermore having different people spoil your child and tempt them with different food can only help eating and maintaining weight.

MEDICAL ISSUES

In order to successfully diagnose Crohn's Disease several different tests will likely be needed as Crohn's has similar symptoms to several other conditions.

Initially, after first falling ill, you will most likely to see your GP several times as they try to establish any pattern to your child's symptoms and to explore any contributing causes. These include our GP your diet and eliminating the effects of recent travel or of the use of any over the counter medications or any other condition such as food poisoning.

Your GP should also carry out a series of standard tests in order to evaluate your child's more general state of health:
   Checking pulse
   Blood pressure
   Measuring temperature for fever
   Examining the abdomen looking for signs of tenderness or pain.
   Measuring height and weight

You may want to get into the habit of keeping regular records of your child's weight gain and loss as it is a very good indicator of how their Crohn's is behaving. By keeping track of this you can increase your own awareness of their general state of health rather than merely relying on what they admit to you.

It is likely that your GP will also arrange a series of blood tests which can be used to assess several things. Firstly they can be used to see if your child has any infections. They also can be used to see if your child is malnourished. If this is the case they will likely be anaemic. Finally a blood test can show the levels of inflammation in the body. When Crohn's Disease is active these levels of inflammation are likely to rise and so this is a good indicator of the disease's activity.

Blood tests are something that you and your child are going to have to undergo with a reasonable degree of regularity and so later in this section we will further explore some mechanisms for dealing with this potentially stressful test.

Due to the symptoms your child is currently experiencing you may be asked to provide a stool sample; some poop in a jar in layman's terms; and this can be used to check for blood or mucus being excreted. A stool sample has several functions such as helping rule out the possibility that the symptoms are being caused by a parasitic infection. As for actually collecting this sample you will usually be gifted with a tiny sample pot that seems frankly way too small for the task at hand. My best advice would be to keep a sense of humour about this and I guess be creative with the collection.

Once a blood and stool sample have been provided, it is likely that your GP will refer to a gastroenterologist who can evaluate the results of your child's tests and then discuss them with you. If the gastroenterologist deems it necessary you will be put forward for one of several complex tests which will allow a more complete and accurate diagnosis. You should be warned ahead of time that some of these are pretty darned unpleasantly invasive and as the parent it will fall on you to help to get your child through this bad period.

Blood Tests and Needles

Since your child has fallen ill, needles and blood tests are unfortunately something that you and your child are now going to have to come to terms with. The key here is simply to ensure that the whole experience is as un-traumatic as possible. As is the case for most people having a blood test needs to become a fairly unspectacular and stress free event.

Some children however are not okay with needles. For these children and their parents, these regular blood tests can be a highly stressful event. The unfortunate thing about a scared child is that they are beyond rationality and beyond bribery. Offers of rewards for good behaviour just don't work.

For you as a parent, having a hysterical child screaming in terror, swearing at anyone in earshot and trying to kick the poor nurse actually performing the test, can undoubtedly be embarrassing. The important thing to remember is to stay calm. So with this in mind here are some tips and tricks that I have come across that should hopefully allow you to avoid a situation where both you and two bulky male nurses have to sit on and pin your child down every time a blood test is required. Trust me; whilst pinning the kid down may get the job done, its not really any fun for anyone involved. And I was that child scared stiff of needles so I speak from bitter experience.

My first tip here is to try and minimize the time spent in the waiting room with your child. Any time spent in that room is time to sit and wallow and think about nothing but what's coming. Forty-five minutes to an hour and a half is a long time to sit and think about the tip of that needle. Fortunately this can usually be minimized with a little forward planning and a little creative thought. Your first best bet would be to have a word with your doctor and see if it is possible to arrange for fast track blood tests to be taken instead. In effect here what you are asking is to jump the queue but in their interests and those of the other patients your child is liable to unnerve as well as yours.

If you are sent to a blood test unit where you take a numbered ticket and wait, it is usually possible to have a quiet chat and ask if you can take your number and then nip to the shops with your child to grab a magazine and a snack or something. Again here the goal is simply to minimize the time spent sat in a waiting room. In my experience the departments are usually fairly helpful with stuff like this, particularly if this is not the first time the two of you have been there.

My next tip revolves around distracting the child whilst the actual blood test is happening. A really good way of doing this is with either an MP3 player, a gaming device, some head phones or an iPad. The idea here that the child is somewhat removed from the room whilst the actual test is happening. In an ideal world you can get them watching a show or listening to a song in the waiting room and then walk in and have them hold out their hand without ever taking their eyes off of the screen or taking off their headphones. Once they are familiar with the procedure this is a great way of doing things and is still how I tackle blood tests to this day.

Next we will address the option of numbing creams and sprays. These are great although they can pose a particular problem if of the type where you need to wait for 30 to 45 minutes so they really do numb the area. Fortunately this is not a problem with numbing sprays where an instant icy mist is sprayed onto the area to numb it. Since this takes next to no time it is an excellent idea and is something you can almost always buy over the counter in a chemists shop so that you always have it to hand when needed.

Unfortunately it needs to be acknowledged that even with all these tips and tricks, some children, such as I was are genuinely so terrified of needles that there will seem to be no consoling them. Steel yourself because it has to be seen through.

Colonoscopy

Crohn's disease can appear anywhere along the gastrointestinal tract; pretty much anywhere between the mouth and the rectum. As such there are several types of scans you are likely to encounter when getting your diagnosis.

The first test we will be looking at is a colonoscopy. This test allows an examination of the inside of your child's colon. In order to achieve this, a tool called an endoscope is used. This is a long flexible tube which has a camera and a light on the end and it is used to transmit images to a screen, allowing the colon to be examined for inflammation and also to judge the severity of any observed inflammation. The endoscope can be fitted with a selection of different surgical tools which can be used to take a number of small samples from different sections of the digestive system. This is called a biopsy. This tissue sample can then be examined under a microscope after the procedure and your medical team will hopefully be able to confirm a number of the cell changes which are known to occur in cases of Crohn's Disease.

The actual procedure itself involves passing the endoscope through the rectum and then threading it up into the colon. Now as tests go this sounds highly unpleasant but fortunately the patient is pretty heavily sedated and speaking from experience you will remember next to none of it. As such I would probably say that this is one of the less unpleasant tests involved in testing for Crohn's Disease, although the preparation required before the test is pretty nasty and is worth taking some time to discuss.

In order for a colonoscopy to work and for clear images to be provided it is necessary for the bowel to be cleared out pretty much completely. This is done approximately 24 hours before the test. Usually this involves a selection of preparation drugs selected by your medical team and the selection can vary according to the team's preferences. More often than not a strong laxative will be involved and apart from the obvious symptoms this will cause, it can potentially also give rise to some pretty strong stomach cramps.

During this process your child will not be allowed to eat. Usually the medications will be administered at around midday so I would recommend that you try and get a good breakfast on board if you can. This will likely improve their mood through a pretty unpleasant day.

Unfortunately this is a procedure that you will be likely to have to go through at least every couple of years but I can help to arm you with some tips to make this ride a little bit easier.

Firstly you are allowed to drink several kinds of drinks during the day and after the drugs have been administered. Now some departments have different preferences on what you are and aren't allowed to drink, but my preference on what to drink is some good quality apple juice. As a clear liquid it won't mess up the quality of the images taken and so you can drink as much as you want. I will usually drink between two and three litres of juice on a day like this. Juice has plenty of sugar and so will help keep the worst of the hunger pains at bay and I find it helps keep my mood up. Since your child will have to drink plenty of fluids anyways to help flush out their system, having a drink you enjoy certainly helps.

My second tip may not be that relevant for your child's first colonoscopy. However as each successive one occurs and you become more familiar with the preparatory procedures and the team treating you, the option can arise to do the necessary preparation meds at home and then travel to the hospital for the procedure in the morning to have the colonoscopy done. I hasten to note that this is at your medical team's discretion but it is a request I have not had denied over recent years. The advantages of being at home in a more familiar, comfortable environment for a preparation day are obvious, although some of the simplest benefits such as having access to your own private toilet, which can really make a big difference in making the day more bearable, are of course achievable in a sympathetic and well-equipped hospital environment too.

Barium X-Rays

A Barium x-ray is pretty similar to a regular one except that prior to the scan a chalky white fluid called barium is administered. This can be either orally or rectally depending upon the area being scanned. If administered orally this is called an Upper GI series and it involves drinking the barium. This is admittedly not pleasant, but it is not that terrible either.

The purpose of the barium is to flow through the intestines making them visible upon the x-ray film, making the identification of problem areas easier.

Wireless Capsule Endoscopy

This is a relatively new type of test which frankly is rather clever. It involves swallowing a small capsule which is about the size of a large vitamin tablet. The capsule contains a small camera which will work its way through the small intestine transmitting images to a recording device which can be carried around. Don't worry; the external device is pretty small and can be worn on a belt or in a small backpack so it won't really restrict your child in anyway. After a couple of days the capsule will be passed as a stool. You won't have to retrieve it, thank goodness. It's disposable so no dirty jobs here.

The images are then transferred from the recording device to a computer so they can be reviewed. This test is pretty new and so availability is somewhat limited, but information is power and so you can most definitely bring this up with your consultant. If ever there was a right time to be a pushy parent, this might be it.

MRE and CT Scans

MRE and CTE Scans are increasingly in use by doctors treating people with Crohn's. As such your little team will be likely to encounter them at some point. This is because they can be especially helpful in locating where the disease is active and where any problem areas are. Your doctor may also be able to identify any areas of the intestine that have narrowed or ulcers which are present.

MRE stands for magnetic resonance enterography. An MRE scan can be used to examine the small intestine of people suspected of having Crohn's Disease. The actual scan itself is for the most part absolutely fine. It involves your child being put in an MRI machine. Magnetic fields and radio waves are then used to produce detailed images of the small intestine. It is worth noting that this can take a bit of time and so some people may find themselves becomes very bored or claustrophobic. One involves falling asleep and the other can lead to panic. Just make sure your child knows that despite the machinery for this test being a little bit loud, it is completely okay and no harm will come to them.

Unfortunately for the scan to take place the patient is required to drink a liquid known as a contrasting agent. I cannot lie: this stuff is disgusting and you will be faced with two options. The first is to grit your teeth, get through it and get the test done. The other approach is to have a naso-gastric tube placed in your child's nose which leads to the small intestine. The contrast agent is then pushed down the tube, pretty much bypassing the need to actually drink the stuff. I have done both and have to say that both suck and this is probably the worst test you will go through. But getting a tube stuck up your nose is really so unpleasant that I would recommend you avoid it if you can.

Next up there are CT scans, which also involve a contrasting agent but instead of taking images with magnetic fields and radio waves, x-rays are used instead. These produce detailed images of the pelvis and abdomen. For the technically minded CT stands for Computerised Tomography.

Ultrasound

Since you have presumably already had at least had one child if you're reading this, I can reasonably safely assume that this is a test you are familiar with. But just in case I will quickly walk you through it. Basically this test involves some cold jelly being placed on your child's tummy and then a scan of the area with a handheld scanner deployed by a radiographer. This test is entirely painless and non-invasive. Possibly this is one of the tests you will actually enjoy. View this as a good opportunity to enjoy your time together, since you are together and since there's nothing unpleasant happening, you might as well make the most of it.

Medication

Unfortunately there is currently no known cure for Crohn's Disease. If however your child is experiencing moderate to severe symptoms then it can be said that they have "active disease". In the event that your child's Crohn's can be considered active then treatment will usually involve medication and in more extreme cases surgery may be considered as an option. Speaking generally there three main goals of treatment and these are set out below.

The first of these goals is to induce what is known as remission. Remission is a length of time where the child is not actively experiencing any symptoms. This goal focuses upon symptom management. That is: using medications to limit or completely stop the symptoms of the disease.
The second goal of treatment is to maintain this period of remission and extend it as long as possible.
The third main goal of treatment for a child is to attempt to promote normal, healthy growth and development as much as possible.

Normally your child's treatment will be provided by a wide range of healthcare professionals and the first order for you as the parent is to ensure that you know who everybody is, what their job is and how they fit into the picture of your child's treatment plan.

Steroids

More often than not, the first treatment offered to you will be steroids, the goal of this being to reduce the inflammation which is causing many of the worst symptoms of the disease.

Some examples include Prednisolone tablets or Budesonide. Practically speaking these medications do not present too much of a problem and once the child is familiar with having to take pills it is one of the easier medications to administer and maintain.

Medications such as these are often effective in reducing the symptoms of Crohn's disease but they can have significant side effects.

Some of the more common of these side effects will include:
    Weight gain
    Swelling of the face
    Increased vulnerability to infections
    Osteoporosis, which is a weakening of the bones (which may leave the patient vulnerable to breaks in the future).

Due to the nature of these side effects, the dose of these drugs which is being administered will be closely monitored so that when symptoms begin to reduce the dosage can gradually be reduced as well.

Liquid Diet

Because maintaining normal growth and development in a child is a particularly important concern, you may also be offered a special liquid diet as an initial treatment.

This involves a liquid which will replace your child's normal sources of nutrition, food, for a number of months. You will be expected to make the liquid up yourself at home from a tin of powder once you are familiar with it and your child will not be able to eat normally during this time.

This liquid diet will have the aim of reducing the stress placed on the gut and allowing it to heal while the treatment is on-going whilst ensuring that your child is getting all the nutrients they require for normal growth.

Practically speaking this is one of the more difficult medications to deal with and it is worth taking some time to help you as the parent understand them. Hopefully by doing so you can better understand some of the difficulties your child will be facing and help to address them.

There are a number of issues commonly faced by those using a liquid diet revolving around both taste and practical issues.

Taste is the biggest long-term obstacle to successful use of a liquid diet. Simply put, the available liquid diets are at best an acquired taste. Fortunately they do now come in a variety of flavours but none the less they do take a bit of getting used to. Patience is probably your best ally here and once some time passes your child will at least get used to it and maybe even grow to love it. I did eventually, although I was thoroughly aware of how odd that fact was.

Then there are all the practical issues around pre-planning and preparation. Being tied to consuming a liquid diet is quite restricting and it impacts require on most aspects of your daily routine. The more on top of this you are, the easier it is for the child who actually has to drink the stuff.

You will need to foster a positive relationship with the school your child is attending. The goal is to promote an environment where, despite the fact that your child is eating in a very different manner to all the other children, this does not disrupt or distress them overly. Personally I was allowed to eat in the main office separately from the other children. I found this the best solution because even once I had got used to the liquid diet, being in a room full of people eating a normal lunch was quite distressing. To put it bluntly the temptation to "cheat on the diet" was overwhelming.

In an ideal world you would not need to worry about your own behaviour affecting your child but the fact of the matter is that having a child on a liquid diet poses a challenge to your own home life. Normal events such as a Sunday roast dinner now completely exclude one member of the family and that can be very hard for them. Now I am not saying that you should abandon these activities entirely but I am encouraging you to communicate to your child that this is on your mind. It will go a long way to making them feel included and will help avoid them feeling isolated and alone in this trying stage.

Further Treatment

If your child's symptoms either flare up twice or more in about a year, or if the symptoms continue once their steroid dosages are reduced, then additional treatment other than that described above may be necessary and further medicines may be prescribed.

One of the first of these that you will be likely to encounter will be immuno-suppressants, which may be combined with the initial treatment. The most common of these medicines which you will be likely to encounter will be Azathioprine or Meracaptopurine. You may also come across a drug called Methotrexate which has similar affects.

Unfortunately these medications can have side effects and they do not necessarily have the same impact on every patient. Accordingly before and during the course of taking these drugs your child will be required to have blood tests fairly regularly to insure that they are not suffering adverse consequences. As with all medications you should discuss the potential side effects with your doctors. Some of the common side effects of immuno-suppressants can be:

    Increased vulnerability to infections
    Nausea and vomiting
    Fatigue, breathless and general feeling of weakness.

Biological Therapies

At some point you may eventually reach the stage where, due to ongoing poor health and severe symptoms, your child will be introduced to biological therapies. This will only happen if both the steroids and immune-suppressants have proven ineffective.

Biological therapies comprise a powerful type of immune-suppressant medications created using naturally occurring antibodies and enzymes. The goal of these biological therapies will be to reduce your child's symptoms to a more manageable level and to induce remission.

Crohn's is admittedly treated differently around the world but in the UK you will encounter two medicines used for this kind of treatment. These are called Adalimumab and Infliximab.

Adalimumab should only be used to treat adults so you don't really need to worry about this one. Infliximab however is used to treat children over six years old and adults so it worth being a little familiar with this drug. Both drugs work by targeting a protein called TNF alpha which is widely regarded as being responsible for the inflammation associated with Crohn's Disease

Infliximab will be given as a drip into the child's arm over a course of a few hours. This is known as an infusion. This will usually take the better part of half a day but this is not always the case and varies from person to person. As far as treatments go it is probably one of the least invasive and stress-free forms of intervention available.

There is however a chance of these drugs causing an allergic reaction which can cause some of the following symptoms. If your child experiences any of these you should contact your medical team and let them know immediately. Your doctor will undoubtedly discuss this in detail but some of the more serious ones to look out for are:
- Itchy skin
- Fever
- Joint and muscle pain
- Swelling of the hands or lips
- Problems swallowing

I have experienced some of these and while admittedly they aren't always pleasant, they were fortunately usually pretty easily dealt with by my medical team.

Surgery

At some point during your treatment plan you may be faced with surgery and this can admittedly be a very scary prospect. Fortunately speaking from experience I can say that it sounds scarier than it is.

The most common type of surgery for people with Crohn's disease is called a re-section. A re-section involves removing the inflamed area of the intestine and stitching the healthy sections back together again. You can rest assured that surgery will not be recommended unless your healthcare team feels that the benefits offered to your child's quality of life outweighs the risks involved.

A re-section will take at least three months to heal and during that time your child will sleep a lot. They will also be pretty weak but this is just an expected result of the surgery. It is important to recognise the required healing time and to be aware that any surgery in the intestinal and rectal areas carries significant risks of subsequent infection and thus of further intervention with antibiotics until healed.

In some cases, your medical team may also recommend an additional procedure called an ileostomy. This is a procedure which will temporarily divert digestive waste away from the inflamed area of the large intestine. The idea behind this is to give the area time to heal.

If an ileostomy is performed then during the operation the ileum, the end of the small intestine, will be disconnected from the colon. A small hole called a stoma will then be made in the abdomen, the ileum will be rerouted through this hole and an external bag can then be attached to the opening to collect waste. The bag will be smell proof so there are no worries there although the number of times per day you need to change the bag can vary.

Once the colon is sufficiently recovered your child can then have another operation to close the stoma and reattach the colon to the small intestine. Usually however this will be several months after the first surgery.

Your medical team will undoubtedly go into more than enough detail about the practicalities of a stoma should one be needed so I won't go on except to say that thankfully a stoma shouldn't really impact on your child's quality of life and once they get used to maintaining it, the impact on their life will be minimal.

All of this sounds pretty complicated and scary, but in my experience, surgery will be a relief when you actually get there. Surgery feels very proactive as a patient. It is nice to get a handle on something that has been spiralling out of control and surgery is a very effective means of doing that.

COMPROMISING TO LIVE

One of the hardest things to do with Crohn's disease is to accept that your child's life will now take a different and more difficult path that their peers. Certain things will be much harder for them than the people around them and some career paths will be closed to them. For example anyone with Crohn's disease is excluded from the armed forces in any capacity and due to it being difficult to maintain a consistent body weight a career as a star athlete is probably not on the cards.

There are however many other options available and you should encourage your child to explore all their interests. Crohn's Disease will make school harder than it is for other children due to the nature of the disease and with relapsing being a constant risk you will find that your child is potentially not the ideal student. It is however more than likely that your child will end up adopting less than the usual approaches to study and you need to be on top of this to ensure that there is not a negative effect on their grades.

Stress is one of the key things that can make Crohn's Disease worse so I would recommend you encourage your child to learn skills that they enjoy and take pleasure in. If any of these turn into a career in the long run that's just an added benefit.

Now to flip things on their head, I would argue that are some pretty awesome benefits to having Crohn's Disease. Firstly by the time your child reaches adulthood he or she will have overcome more challenges than most people face in a lifetime. This will make them strong and able to approach almost any problem in a dynamic manner. Having lived with Crohn's for so many years already there are now very few problems that I feel I couldn't overcome. This is an attitude you should try to foster. Once you have dealt with Crohn's pretty much everything else is easy in comparison.

HOLISTIC SYMPTOM MANAGEMENT

This section will aim to cover some of the more unorthodox ways in which you can help your child feel better when they are suffering a flare up. To clarify, none of the following will treat Crohn's Disease, but what they will do is help your child to relax and make them feel better.

Firstly we have massage therapy. One of the most troubling and annoying symptoms of Crohn's is the presence of stiff muscles and joints. Any effort to alleviate this will be greatly appreciated and can greatly improve the child's outlook. While it is worth noting that this is something you can pay for, it is also one of the few ways in which you can directly help and so you might consider massage a skill worth learning.

Next up we have reflexology. This involves massaging the feet and hands with a series of specific techniques. The idea here being that there are a system of reflex areas in the feet and hands which correspond to the rest of the body and these zones can be manipulated through massage and this will have an effect on the rest of the body.

Now I want to make it clear that these are not treatments for Crohn's Disease but are a proactive means by which you can help your child relax. Furthermore by working with them you can help them to learn how to perform this type of massage on their own. This will give your child a means of helping themselves to wind down and relax, which is a very handy skill to have. I use this technique and I have found it to be a great help when trying to sleep despite pain and discomfort.

CLOSING COMMENTS ON NUTRITION

It is important to understand that for anyone with Crohn's Disease food becomes a pretty complicated issue, both mentally and physically. The most important thing to appreciate is that food can become a scary prospect, one that causes a lot of pain and discomfort. It will be fairly easy for your child to fall into a pattern of avoiding eating whenever possible.

As a parent seeing your child refuse to eat can be hard to make sense of, but understanding why they don't want to eat will go a long way to helping comfort them. Being aware that someone who understands is in their corner is a big deal; it helps them feel normal about their eating habits.

Your child's eating habits may rapidly become quite strange. They may become prone to whole days without eating as well as suffering from odd cravings at unusual times. My theory is that for any one with Crohn's Disease these cravings are ways for their bodies to tell them what they need to eat in order to fulfil their nutritional requirements. With this in mind I would encourage you to indulge these cravings, even if this is just to see them eat something. After all one meal a day is better than none.

KEY TERMS

Biopsy: Removing and then examining a small amount of tissue, with the intention of discovering more about the illness

Diagnosis: A judgement about what a particular illness is, once it has been examined a cause can be identified

Fatigue: Extreme tiredness

Flare Up: A situation in which something suddenly starts or gets much worse

Gastrointestinal tract: This is made up of the stomach and the intestine, which is the long tube food passes through once it leaves the stomach.

Inflammation: A painful and often swollen area of the body

In-patient: This is where someone goes into hospital and stays at least one night to receive treatment

Nausea: The overwhelming sense that you are going to be sick

Out-patient: This is where someone goes into hospital to receive treatment but is not required to stay overnight.

Remission: A period of time when an illness is less severe or is not affecting someone

Ulcer: An open wound on the surface of an organ inside the body. This will not heal naturally.

FURTHER INFORMATION

For UK sufferers
http://www.reddit.com/r/CrohnsDisease/
http://www.crohnsandcolitis.org.uk
http://www.cicra.org/

For American and Canadian sufferers
http://www.ccfa.org
http://www.crohnsandcolitis.ca

For European sufferers
http://www.efcca.org

OTHER HEALTH AND LIFESTYLE BOOKS FROM APS PUBLICATIONS
(see www.andrewsparke.com)

Beating The Banana: Breast Cancer and Me (Helen Pitt)
Changing Lives: The Leaps and Bounds Method (Horsfall & Sparke)
Food and Cancer Prevention (Andrew Sparke)
What I Think About When I Think about Aikido (Mark Peckett)
Your Kid and Crohn's: A Parent's Handbook (William Sparke)

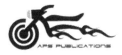

SERVICES FOR ASPIRING WRITERS FROM APS PUBLICATIONS

- You write
- We edit
- We provide cover art
- We publish to Kindle
- You help market your book
- We are highly affordable
- You get at least 50% royalties

Does that sound fair? We exist to help our authors not to exploit them. Contact andrew.sparke@blueyonder.co.uk

Ever since I set up my own publishing imprint and published 'Indie Publishing: The Journey Made Easy' on Kindle to persuade people that DIY is the way to go rather than wasting time chasing elusive agents and even rarer publishing deals, I've had regular approaches from lovely refuseniks who just want to produce a manuscript and have someone else organise their editing and publication. And of course these are time-consuming processes that take you away from the business of writing. So if it helps talk to us because APS Publications can now do it for you. And we help run weekly and monthly writers groups in Birmingham and the Black Country which welcome new joiners.

Look forward to hearing from you,

Andrew Sparke

Manufactured by Amazon.ca
Bolton, ON